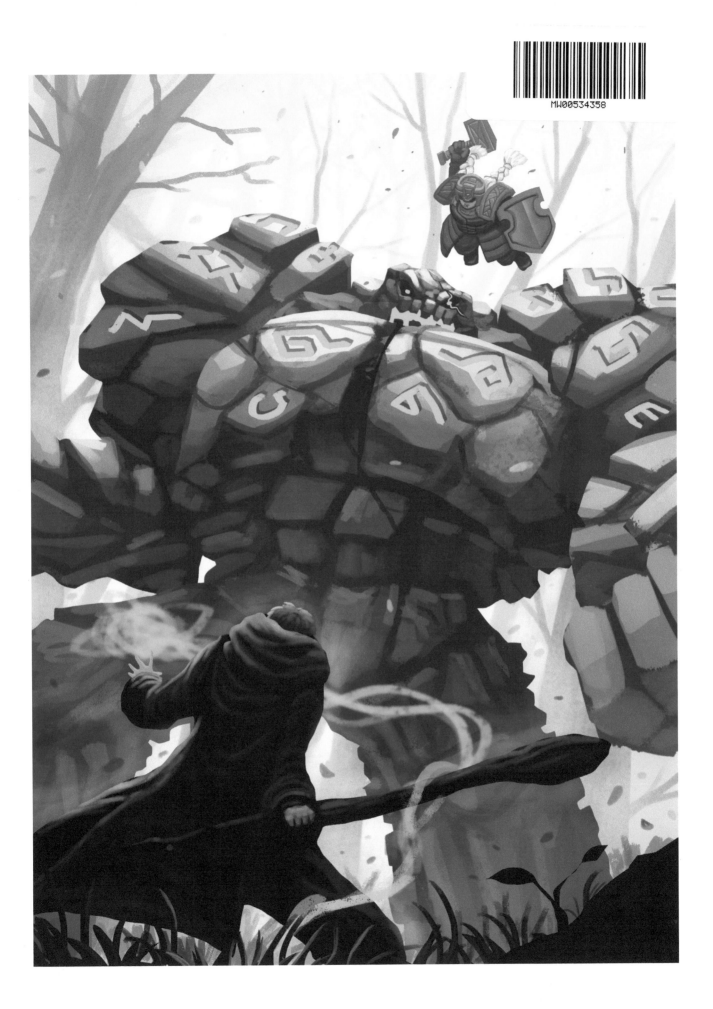

Contents

Legal Disclaimer

Credits

Authors: Phoenix Grey and Sky Corgan
Illustrators: Wenart Gunadi, Map Creative, El Art, Haosekii Art, r3d_five5, and Simon Zhong
Logo Design: Legend_Designers
Template Design: Nathanaël Roux

INTRODUCTION

 ELCOME TO LEWD DUNGEON ADVENTURES, an adult role-playing game filled with fantasy and fun. Before you go any further, you should know that this book is meant for the Deity's eyes only. Reading it as a Hero will ruin the game for you.

In the following pages, Deities will find details on how to run the scenarios in this campaign. If you have not read the rulebook yet, please go back and do so before beginning the game.

PREPARING FOR GAMEPLAY

Heroes need only come with a character sheet, a willingness to learn, and a great imagination. It is recommended that the Deity read through the campaign before gameplay to know what is coming and how to plan for it.

The following campaign book is divided into 5 mini-adventures. This particular campaign book was designed to be played in 5 sessions, but an ambitious Hero and Deity can power through as many of the adventures as they'd like.

REQUIRED PROPS

This campaign requires the following props:

- 4 Candles
- Ice
- Blindfold

If you do not have candles, any four sources of light can be substituted, such as lamps.

CAMPAIGN OVERVIEW

Following the passing of the Kegel Empire's Grand Master Mage, Nhedam Hussa, Emperor Geo Crapflare sent out a missive to The Copper Cove School of Magic to request their dean, Famuhlel Pehe, to become Nhedam's replacement. Famuhlel's presence was required at the palace immediately, forcing her to leave her belongings behind to be delivered at a later date.

Unfortunately, the caravan escorting her things was set upon by bandits, and five crates of irreplaceable magic items were stolen. Knowing what would be at stake if the crates fell into the wrong hands, Famuhlel had the foresight to place tracking magic on each one.

Because of the nature of the items, she is requesting the help of a Cummancer to retrieve them. Arming the Hero with a list of locations where the crates could be found, she warns that whoever took them will likely use strong magic and fierce force to keep them from returning to their owner.

At the start of the campaign, read the text box:

Grand Master Mage Famuhlel Pehe was having her belongings transported from The Copper Cove School of Magic to Kegel Palace when the caravan was set upon by bandits.

Five crates of incredibly rare magical items were stolen, and she fears they might fall into the wrong hands if not retrieved quickly. Due to the nature of the contents of the crates, Famuhlel needs the special skills of a Cummancer to complete the job.

Luckily, she had the foresight to place tracking magic on the crates before they were stolen, so she knows the location of each one but not the dangers that may await.

She gives you a map marked with the location of each crate as well as a number order for which they should be retrieved, telling you to not ask questions or pry into the contents of the crates. If you can retrieve all five, you will be rewarded handsomely for your efforts.

STARTING THE ADVENTURE

If this is the first time your Hero has played Lewd Dungeon Adventures, have them start by introducing their character. Some players may choose to create an entire backstory for their character. They should be encouraged to explain it in detail.

Next, you can explain the basis of Lewd Dungeon Adventures, that you are a Deity of sexual energy that has blessed them with your favor. Because of your partnership, they have been bestowed with special sex magic that will cause them to be sought out across the land to complete quests that can only be undertaken by one with their skills and knowledge. With your blessing, they are now known as a Cummancer.

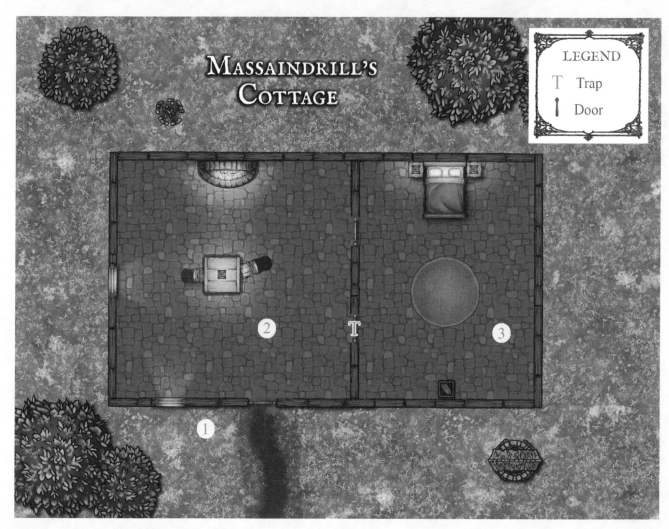

SCENARIO 1: AN UNEXPECTED PARTY

The first crate is located in the home of Massaindrill Highsun, a witch and rival to Famuhlel Pehe. A professor at The Copper Cove School of Magic, she knew that Famuhlel's belongings would be in commute and orchestrated the robbery, taking what she wanted and selling the rest to other unscrupulous mages of the wizarding underbelly.

The journey to the first location takes the Hero through Peaceful Cedar Covert and up to the top of a hill where Massaindrill's cottage stands in seclusion amidst a few scattered trees.

Multiple Hero Modification: For this entire scenario, keep the number of monsters the same no matter how many Heroes are in the party.

AREA 1: OUTSIDE THE COTTAGE

Upon the Hero's arrival, read the text box below:

> When you reach the top of the hill marked on your map, the forest gives way to a small wooden cottage. The sound of multiple voices reaches you before the structure comes into view, though they're muffled through the walls.
>
> A window to the left of the door clearly displays a host of people inside, standing around chatting. It appears that the occupants are having a party.

The only thing of note in front of the cottage is a medium-sized stone well. Looking inside, the well is so deep that the Hero cannot see the bottom. Should they lower the basket to check the contents of the well, they will only bring water back up.

Behind the cottage is a small fire pit, though the only thing in it is ash. Otherwise, there is nothing else around the cottage aside from the footpaths that Massaindrill and her gobblin companion have made.

Magic has been cast on the window to make it look like people are inside, but it's just an illusion.

If the Hero uses UV Light around the cottage, they will be able to tell that the cottage's windows have been enchanted.

Have the Hero make a Hard roll to check for footprints. If they roll a 5 or higher, let them know that they only see two sets of footprints in front of the cottage, one set belonging to a human and the other to a gobblin.

Should the Hero try to listen to what the people are saying, have them roll a d6. Regardless of the outcome, the voices are too muffled for them to pick out any bits of conversation. This is part of Massaindrill's spell. The people aren't saying anything at all, simply muttering inaudibly to make it sound like they are speaking.

A Hero who explores around the cottage will not find anything helpful. While another window on the left side of the cottage displays the same image of people talking inside, there are no other entrances to the building.

The Hero will only be able to enter Massaindrill's cottage by force. Despite all the people they see in the window, if the Hero tries to get their attention, they are ignored. This should be the first hint that something is amiss.

If the Hero knocks on the door, no one comes to answer. Should they try to open the door, they will find it locked. The Hero now has three choices for entering the cottage.

They can use their lockpicks. The lock on the cottage door is simple and can be picked with an Easy roll of 3 or higher.

They can use force. This is a bit more difficult to do, requiring a Hard roll of 5 or higher.

The third and easiest option is to break the window and enter that way. Breaking the window requires nothing more than a blunt object and a Very Easy roll of 2 or higher.

It is up to the Deity's discretion as to whether they will allow the Hero to roll multiple times for the same method of entry or force them to seek another way inside. Should the Hero fail two of the three methods of entry, the third method will automatically succeed.

AREA 2: INSIDE THE COTTAGE

As soon as the Hero breaches the cottage, read the text box below:

> Despite the vision that you saw through the window, the inside of the cottage is void of life aside from a single gobblin standing with its club in hand.
>
> A quick glance around shows a fire crackling in a fireplace across from the front door. Set in the middle of the room is a square wooden table with two chairs. Sitting atop it, a lantern provides additional illumination to the otherwise empty space.
>
> There are two doors on the eastern wall, both shut. However, you cannot be concerned with them right now because the gobblin is ready to fight!

Once they enter the cottage, the Hero will be set upon by Massaindrill's companion. An outcast among its kind, this gobblin was captured by the mages of The Copper Cove School of Magic and Massaindrill has since taken it under her wing, using it to test various potions in return for giving it food and shelter.

While not fiercely loyal to her, it will defend the cottage until its Health Points are reduced to 3 or below, at which point it will beg for its life.

This particular gobblin speaks very broken Common. Its disposition is fearful and distrusting.

Should the Hero try to seduce the gobblin, it will submit in an attempt to buy Massaindrill time to come up with a plan of action. She currently resides in area 3 and can hear everything going on outside of her room.

If the Hero wants to seduce the gobblin, set a timer for 5 minutes. The Hero must engage in rough, fast sex with the gobblin (played by you) in any position the gobblin chooses. Once the timer goes off, the gobblin will be satiated. If combat has not yet taken place, it will ensue afterward. However, if the gobblin's Health Points have already been reduced to 3 or under, the gobblin will request to leave following the act of intimacy.

Should the Hero question the gobblin about the crate's location, it will pretend not to know what they are talking about. However, the gobblin is well aware that the crate is in the next room with Massaindrill.

If the gobblin is asked what is in the other room, it will say it's not allowed in there. Should the Hero ask if anyone else is inside the cottage, the gobblin will lie and say it does not know.

Have the Hero make a Normal roll. With a successful roll of 4 or higher, the Hero will be able to tell that the gobblin is lying due to the sweat gathering on its brow and the fact that it keeps looking nervously toward the left.

Threatening the gobblin will produce no further information.

It is up to the Hero whether they want to allow the gobblin to escape or not. There is no reward for letting the gobblin live, but the Hero will acquire a firestarter as loot if they defeat the gobblin.

Once the gobblin has been dealt with, the Hero will be free to explore the room. A Hero who uses the UV Light spell will be able to tell that the southeastern door is false and a trap.

GOBBLIN

Roll to Hit: 4+
Health Points: 7

Traits: Night Vision
Sex Style: Rough and Quick
Languages: Common, Gobblin

Description: Yes, the name is spelled right. Standing five feet tall with squat bodies, olive-green skin, and pointed ears, gobblins are known for fornicating with whatever creatures they can get their hands on.

ATTACKS

Club. Melee Weapon Attack: one target. Hit: (1d4) damage.

Sling. Ranged Weapon Attack: one target. Hit: (1d4) ranged damage.

Southeastern Door: Should the Hero try to open this door, they will fall victim to a spell that causes them to shrink down to half their size, reducing their remaining Health Points by half rounded up. Any Roll for Damage they make will also be divided by half. If the result is an uneven number, round up. This effect remains in place until the Hero's next death.

Northeastern Door: This door has been rigged as a trap in a different way. The second that the Hero tries to open it, a cast of crabs comes out from around it, immediately engaging them in combat. Massaindrill will shut the door once the crabs have been unleashed, buying herself more time to come up with a plan.

The cast of crabs cannot be seduced or reasoned with. Their stat block is below:

CAST OF CRABS

Roll to Hit: 3+
Health Points: 12

Traits: Night Vision
Sex Style: None
Languages: None

Description: Each the size of a human hand, there are a dozen crabs in this cast. They are adept climbers and go straight for your pubes.

ATTACKS

Pube Yank. Weaponless Attack: one target. *Hit:* (1d12) damage. When its Health Points are reduced by half, Pube Yank does (1d6) damage.

Once the cast of crabs has been defeated, the Hero will be free to enter the northeastern door.

Death: If the Hero dies in this room, they will respawn outside of Massaindrill's cottage.

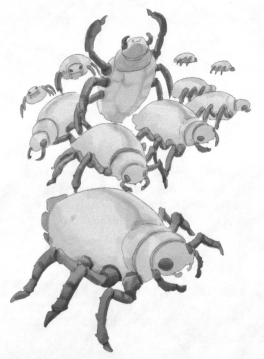

Area 3: Massaindrill's Bedroom

The northeastern door leads to Massaindrill's bedroom, where she's been patiently waiting, hoping that one of her traps or monsters would take care of the Hero before they got this far. Unfortunately, for her, she was wrong. Now, she must put her final plan into action.

When the Hero enters this room, read the following text box:

This room appears to be a bedroom. A queen size bed sits a few yards away. Lanterns on nightstands illuminate the windowless area, and a large circular green rug covers the stone floor.

Standing before a large wooden crate to the south is a scantily clad woman wearing a purple witch's hat. She has her back to you and sighs heavily. When she turns around, her violet eyes linger on the crate for a moment before landing on you.

"I know what you're here for," she begins in a serious tone. "How about we make a deal?"

Massaindrill doesn't want to fight, but she will if she has to. In an attempt to keep the crate, she will offer two things to the Hero in exchange for them walking away. The first is her body. Because she knows she's in a dire predicament, Massaindrill will be willing to please the Hero however they choose. However, the Hero must agree to a blood oath before doing so. If they take Massaindrill up on her offer, they will not be able to leave with the crate.

If the Hero refuses the first offer, Massaindrill will next offer the Hero a Potion of Enlargement. The potion will double the Hero's size. As a result, their Hit Points will double as will the amount of damage they do when they Roll for Damage. Any skill roll involving strength will also be doubled, and Critical Hits will be worth 4x damage. The effects last until the Hero's next death.

Again, the deal requires a blood oath that will result in the Hero being unable to retrieve the crate. Should the Hero take Massaindrill up on either deal, they can still complete the rest of the scenarios, but Famuhlel will see through any lie they come up with as to why they did not retrieve the first crate and will deny them a reward at the end of the campaign for their dishonesty.

If a blood oath is made, the Hero will lose a single Health Point from a cut to their palm needed to collect the blood for the oath, but they will be able to leave Massaindrill's cottage peaceably. However, if they refuse both offers, combat will ensue.

Before this happens, the Hero may wish to question Massaindrill about the crate's contents and how she came to be in possession of it. She will deny any involvement in the robbery, saying that someone sold it to her. While Massaindrill is a great witch, she's not a very good liar. Have the Hero roll a Normal skill check to see if she's telling the truth. On a successful roll of 4 or higher, the Hero will have a pretty good feeling that she's being dishonest. If asked what's in the crate, Massaindrill will lie by omission, saying that she hasn't been able to open it yet. Strong magic keeps the crate sealed, though Massaindrill is most certainly aware of its contents.

MASSAINDRILL HIGHSUN

Roll to Hit: 4+
Health Points: 19

Traits: None
Sex Style: Compliant
Languages: Common, Gobblin, Amazonian

Description: A Copper Cove School of Magic professor, this witch dabbles in dark sex magic.

ATTACKS

Bad Touch. Unlimited Spell: one target. *Hit:* (1d8) ranged damage.

Reflective Barrier. Limited Spell: self

Massaindrill is very powerful and is not meant to be defeated the first time around. She can cast two spells, Bad Touch and Reflective Barrier. The stat blocks for both are below.

BAD TOUCH
Requirements: Must be able to move hands.
Type: Unlimited
Range: Ranged
Description: Ethereal hands form to touch a target within view in every uncomfortable way imaginable. The sheer feeling of disgust does 1d8 damage to the soul.

REFLECTIVE BARRIER
Requirements: Must be able to speak.
Type: Limited
Range: Self
Description: A thick rubber barrier forms around the caster, protecting them from 3 damage and reflecting that damage back on the attacker. The effects of this spell last for the entire combat, and casting it requires an action.

Massaindrill will only use Bad Touch until her Health Points have been reduced by half, at which point she will cast Reflective Barrier. She only has one Limited spell available, so will only be able to cast the spell once. After that, she will return to using Bad Touch until the end of the fight.

Once Massaindrill is defeated, the Hero will be able to take the Potion of Englargement from her. If the Hero uses the Potion of Enlargement while under the effects of the shrinking spell, they will simply return to their normal size with their normal stats, as the two will counteract each other.

The crate is also now theirs for the taking. Though it is heavy, it takes no special equipment to remove it.

Searching the room will prove fruitless as there is nothing else of value to pillage. Should the Hero try to open any of the crates throughout this campaign, they will take 1d4 damage, as the crates are protected by magic meant to keep bandits out. It is not possible for the crates to be opened by the Hero.

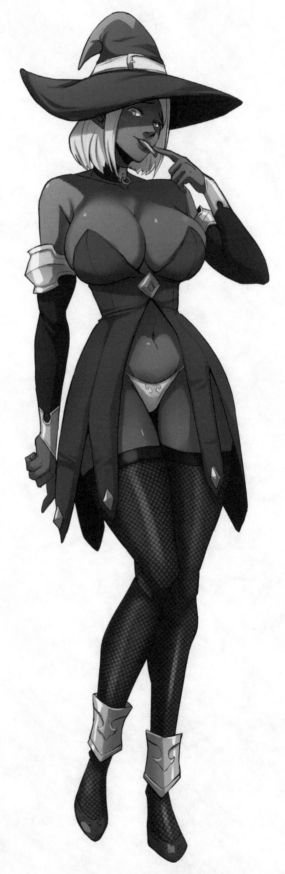

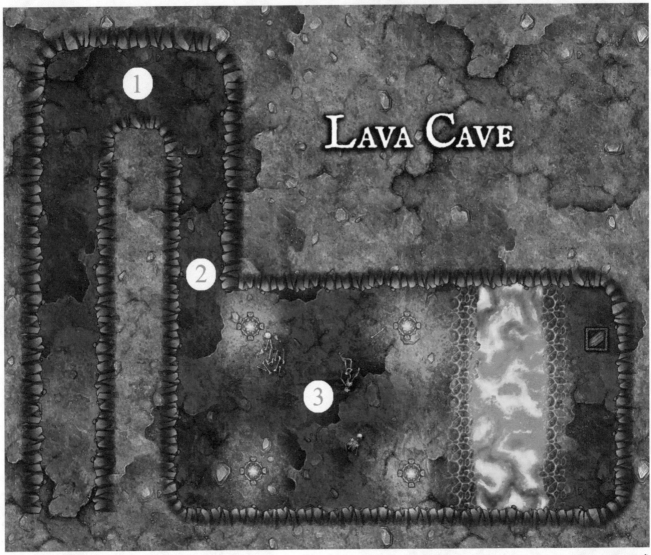

SCENARIO 2: A TALE OF FIRE

The second of the five crates was sold to Daerthrun Peenhandle, a dwarven fire mage. He took the crate deep below the earth's surface to a cave to protect it while he went away on a personal matter.

Unfortunately, Daerthrun was followed, so the Hero will have competition in retrieving the crate.

AREA 1: CAVE ENTRANCE

Start the scenario by reading the text box below:

> The next location on your map brings you to a natural cave entrance. Several sets of footprints lead in and out of the narrow tunnel, though you can see no light coming from inside.

Any Hero wanting to enter the cave that does not have an item that grants them night vision will be forced to light a torch before entering. There is plenty of dry wood around with which to do this. Once they enter the cave, read the text box:

> You descend several hundred feet before the tunnel turns sharply to the right. As soon as you round the corner, you come face to face with a sex cultist.

This sex cultist is standing guard while his buddy further down in the cave is busy trying to figure out how to get to the crate.

SEX CULTIST

Roll to Hit: 4+
Health Points: 9

Traits: None
Sex Style: Mutual
Languages: Common

Description: A humanoid hoping to gain the favor of a Deity by actively pursuing the knowledge of sex magic.

ATTACKS

Whip. Melee Weapon Attack: one target. *Hit:* (1d4) damage.

Blowgun. Ranged Weapon Attack: one target. *Hit:* (1d4) ranged damage.

Multiple Heroes Modification: If there is more than one Hero in your party, add an extra sex cultist for each additional Hero.

Have the Hero make a Very Hard roll. It will take a successful roll of 6 for the sex cultist not to have heard the Hero coming.

If the sex cultist heard the Hero coming, they will automatically take their combat turn first. No roll for Turn Order is necessary.

If the Hero tries to seduce the sex cultist, they will comply, trying to buy their friend more time to get to the crate. Sex cultists have a mutual sex style, which means they will couple with the Hero in whatever manner they both find agreeable.

Once the act is complete, the sex cultist will go on the offensive, picking back up in combat where they left off or initiating it otherwise.

Death: If the Hero dies in this area, they will respawn outside the cave.

AREA 2: BEFORE THE CHAMBER

After the Hero defeats the sex cultist, read the text box below:

> Not long after continuing down the tunnel, you begin to see light in the distance. About fifty feet further, another sex cultist is standing facing what appears to be an opening to a chamber. Fixated by whatever he's staring at, he does not notice you until you are almost upon him.

This sex cultist is the brains of the operation and most definitely not a fighter. If the Hero tries to initiate combat, he will immediately plead to be spared. Realizing that his companion has been slain, his priorities will quickly switch from retrieving the crate to escaping the tunnel with his life. As a bargaining chip, he will offer to teach the Hero the Unlimited spell Splash Guard as well as share all the information he knows about what lies ahead.

Multiple Hero Modification: Regardless of how many Heroes are in the party, there is only one sex cultist in this area.

What the sex cultist knows: Should the Hero be merciful, the sex cultist will quickly spill that he saw Daerthrun Peenhandle bring the crate deep into the cave. He will also inform the Hero that the dwarf is a fire mage and has cast some type of powerful fire magic to protect the crate from other thieves. The cultist will divulge that he has tried going into the next chamber but that the fog is so thick that he could barely see an inch in front of his face, and every time he's entered the chamber, he was attacked by a fire monster. He is unsure about the exact location of the crate or how to deal with the fog or the monster.

This sex cultist can also be seduced, though no additional benefits will be gained from it.

The stat box for Splash Guard is as follows:

SPLASH GUARD
Requirements: Must be able to speak.
Type: Unlimited
Range: Self
Description: You make an upward wave of your hands, causing a thin sheet of plastic to rise before you. The splash guard will protect you against half of any incoming magic damage you would have otherwise taken from an attack until the end of your next turn. It does not protect against melee damage. This spell must be cast before the damage is received.

Death: If the Hero dies in this area, they will respawn in area 1.

AREA 3: THE FIRE CHAMBER

Read the text box below once the Hero chooses to enter the chamber:

> Peering into the seemingly large chamber, the fog is so thick that you can only see about ten feet in front of you. There's a faint orange glow to the east that appears to be stationary. The cave wall continues southward, and you see a less prominent light in the distance.
>
> As soon as you step into the chamber, you notice the heat in the air. No doubt, there is fire somewhere nearby. Your best guess is that it's coming from the source of the glow.
>
> Bones of a humanoid litter the ground near the threshold of your vision's reach.

Because of the Hero's limited vision, casting UV Light or Grabby Hands will not reveal anything in this area.

If the Hero ventures further into the room, regardless if it's toward the sources of light or elsewhere, they are set upon by a flame of passion.

Multiple Heroes Modification: If there is more than one Hero in your party, do not add any additional flames of passion. This monster gets stronger each time it's defeated, and it will need to be defeated multiple times to dispel the magic protecting the crate.

After the first time the flame of passion is defeated, read the text box:

> Upon defeating the flame of passion, the fog suddenly clears, and you can see the sources of the room's illumination and where all the heat is coming from.
>
> To the east is a river of lava, creating a barrier between you and a small patch of land that the crate rests upon. The river is far too wide for you to ever hope to jump it. Behind the crate, red glowing rocks are lodged into the cave wall, forming a jagged language that you cannot decipher.
>
> In all four corners of the chamber are large brass braziers with fires burning brightly in each one. The two closest to the lava river are on your side.

FLAME OF PASSION

Roll to Hit: 4+
Health Points: 4

Traits: Immune to melee damage. Can only receive damage from magic.
Sex Style: None
Languages: None

Description: Created by fire magic, the flame of passion burns brightly until its purpose is fulfilled. Standing at the height of the average human male, you believe you can see bodies entwined in coitus in the dancing red flames.

ATTACKS

Burn of Love. Weaponless Attack: one target. *Hit:* (1d4) ranged damage.

Daerthrun Peenhandle has enchanted the crate so that it is immovable unless all four braziers have been extinguished.

While the Hero cannot read the language written on the wall, their Deity can. These are the instructions on how to dispel the magic that Daerthrun put in place to protect the crate.

This is a Special Scenario.

XXX – The Deity decodes the ancient language, telling the Hero that they must perform sex magic to dispel the spell and make the lava passable. To do this, they must first have sex in the middle of the room, between the four braziers. The act of intimacy can be anything the Hero and their Deity chooses and must be carried out until either the Hero or Deity is satisfied.

Once the first act is complete, the brazier in the northwest corner of the room will become extinguished, channeling its heat into a new flame of passion that will have to be defeated. See the stat box for flame of passion 2 on the following page.

After defeating it, the Hero and their Deity must take to the middle of the room to perform another act of intimacy until satisfaction. Once the act has been completed, the brazier to the southeast will be extinguished, birthing a third flame of passion to life, which will also need to be defeated. Use the stat box for flame of passion 3 for this one.

After the third flame of passion has been defeated, the Hero and their Deity will take to the middle of the room to perform a third act of intimacy to satisfaction, which will extinguish the northeastern brazier. The final and most powerful flame of passion will be born from this. Use the flame of passion 4 stat box.

This will leave one final brazier, which the Hero and Deity will once more need to complete a sex act to satisfaction to extinguish.

Once the final brazier has been extinguished, the lava will dry up, creating firm passable terrain for the Hero to walk across to retrieve the crate.

Required Props: Four candles, one in each corner of the room. Blow out one candle for each brazier extinguished.
Multiple Heroes Modification: If there is more than one Hero in the party, all Heroes may engage in intimacy with the Deity at once. Each Hero engaged simultaneously will snuff out an additional brazier.

> **Example:** Two Heroes and their Deity have a threesome in the middle of the room. When the act is complete, two braziers will be extinguished instead of just one. This will birth two flames of passion into existence. If this is the first sex act to be completed for this special scenario, it will result in a Flame of Passion 2 and a Flame of Passion 3.

Alternatively, the Deity can engage with a different partner for each brazier.

This particular special scenario requires the Deity to be involved in each sex act to extinguish the braziers.

DRINK - The Deity decodes the ancient language, telling the Hero that they must imbibe in a special fire elixir to dispel the spell and make the lava passable. This can be a one-ounce pour of Fireball, Peppermint Schnapps, or any other spicy liquor or liqueur. Alternatively, you can take three drinks of your favorite spicy adult beverage. Bloody Marys, Micheladas, or Jalapeno Margaritas are the perfect choice for this. Both the Hero and their Deity must take a drink to disarm the spell.

Once the first elixir is taken, the brazier in the northwest corner of the room will become extinguished, channeling its heat into a new flame of passion that will have to be defeated. See the stat box for flame of passion 2 below.

After defeating it, the Hero and their Deity must take another shot or round of drinks. Once that is done, the brazier to the southeast will be extinguished, birthing a third flame of passion to life, which will also need to be defeated. Use the stat box for flame of passion 3 for this one.

After the third flame of passion has been defeated, the Hero and their Deity will take a third round of drinks, which will extinguish the northeastern brazier. The final and most powerful flame of passion will be born from this. Use the flame of passion 4 stat block.

This will leave one final brazier left, which the Hero and Deity will once more be required to drink to extinguish.

Once the final brazier has been extinguished, the lava will dry up, creating firm passable terrain for the Hero to walk across to retrieve the crate.

Multiple Heroes Modification: Everyone in the party must drink each time.
BASE – The Deity decodes the ancient language, telling the Hero that they must correctly say an incantation over each brazier, then defeat the monsters that spring forth before moving on to the next. The Hero may say the incantation over any brazier of their choosing. They do not need to be done in any order.

For the first incantation, have the Hero make a Hard roll. On a successful roll of 5 or higher, the brazier extinguishes. On a failed roll, a flame of passion is born, and they will have to defeat it before trying again.

Once the monster is defeated, they may try the roll again. Every time they fail, they must fight another flame of passion until they succeed on the roll and are able to extinguish the brazier.

Then they will move on to the second brazier. This brazier will require a Normal roll of 4 or greater to extinguish. On a failed roll, the Hero must fight and defeat a flame of passion 2. Once it is defeated, they will make the roll again, battling another flame of passion 2 if they fail or moving on to the next brazier if they pass. You can find the stat block for the flame of passion 2 below.

Once they pass the roll for the second brazier, the Hero will move on to the third. To extinguish the third brazier, they will need to make an Easy roll of 3 or greater. Should they fail the roll, they will have to fight a flame of passion 3. The process will continue as with the previous braziers.

To extinguish the fourth brazier, the Hero will have to succeed in a Very Easy roll, rolling a 2 or greater. Otherwise, they will have to face a flame of passion 4. Just like with the previous braziers, a new enemy will spawn every time the Hero fails the roll.

Once the final brazier has been extinguished, the lava will dry up, creating firm passable terrain for the Hero to walk across to retrieve the crate.

Multiple Heroes Modification: If the party chooses, a different Hero may say each incantation.

FLAME OF PASSION 2

Roll to Hit: 4+
Health Points: 6

Traits: Immune to melee damage. Can only receive damage from magic.
Sex Style: None
Languages: None

Description: Created by fire magic, the flame of passion burns brightly until its purpose is fulfilled. Standing at the height of the average human male, you believe you can see bodies entwined in coitus in the dancing red flames.

ATTACKS

Burn of Love. Weaponless Attack: one target. *Hit:* (1d6) ranged damage.

These battles can be intense. Depending on the stamina and preferences of your Hero, now might be a good time to try a hybrid game, mixing the XXX, DRINK, and BASE options between the different braziers. This can also help to make gameplay a bit more diverse.

Once the lava has grown cold, the Hero can retrieve the crate. There is no other loot to be found in this area.

Death: If the Hero dies in this room, they respawn in area 2.

FLAME OF PASSION 3

Roll to Hit: 4+
Health Points: 8

Traits: Immune to melee damage. Can only receive damage from magic.
Sex Style: None
Languages: None

Description: Created by fire magic, the flame of passion burns brightly until its purpose is fulfilled. Standing at the height of the average human male, you believe you can see bodies entwined in coitus in the dancing red flames.

ATTACKS

Burn of Love. Weaponless Attack: one target. *Hit:* (1d8) ranged damage.

FLAME OF PASSION 4

Roll to Hit: 4+
Health Points: 10

Traits: Immune to melee damage. Can only receive damage from magic.
Sex Style: None
Languages: None

Description: Created by fire magic, the flame of passion burns brightly until its purpose is fulfilled. Standing at the height of the average human male, you believe you can see bodies entwined in coitus in the dancing red flames.

ATTACKS

Burn of Love. Weaponless Attack: one target. *Hit:* (1d10) ranged damage.

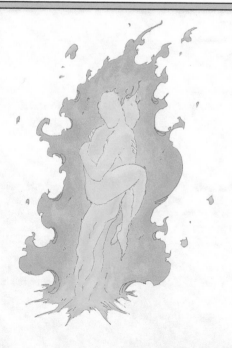

Scenario 3: Guarded by Stone

The third crate was sold to a novice elven earth mage named Jokrana Poplarbirth. Though she's made sure to hide her crate in a hole in the ground, she has mostly decided to rely on hiring thugs and monsters to keep it safe.

There is no map for this scenario.

Area 1: Unpleasant Encounter

Start the scenario by reading the text box below:

> Once again, you find yourself traipsing out into the forest. There's nothing remarkable about the landscape you traversed to get here, mainly consisting of flatland with a few hilly areas.
>
> As you approach the location marked on your map, you see a few game trails, but any footprints around have either been well concealed or are non-existent.

Jokrana has two main lines of defense in place to protect her stolen crate. The first is a dirty bastard she hired to scout the area for intruders. Because of the debauchery that he's regularly involved in, he's rather good at covering his tracks and staying silent in the shadows.

Have the Hero make a Hard roll to detect him. On a successful roll of 5 or higher, the Hero notices the dirty bastard hiding behind a tree before he has a chance to attack. On a failed roll, the dirty bastard earns the element of surprise, granting them the first strike in combat. In this case, no roll for Turn Order is needed.

Multiple Heroes Modification: If there is more than one Hero in your party, add one extra dirty bastard per Hero.

DIRTY BASTARD

Roll to Hit: 4+
Health Points: 13

Traits: None
Sex Style: Porn Roulette
Languages: Common

Description: A humanoid often found at brothels, catcalling people on the streets, and deeply involved in the seedy underbelly of the sex trade.

ATTACKS

Scimitar. *Melee Weapon Attack:* one target. *Hit:* (1d6) damage.

Crossbow. *Ranged Weapon Attack:* one target. *Hit:* (1d6) ranged damage.

The dirty bastard can be seduced, but their tastes are pretty varied. To role-play a sexual encounter with the dirty bastard, go to the porn website of your choice and act out the first video that comes up.

Should the Hero seduce the dirty bastard, they will allow the Hero to pass, mainly out of curiosity to see if the Hero can get past the next obstacle and claim the crate. However, the dirty bastard will fight the Hero on their way back, wanting to take the crate for themselves.

If the Hero questions the dirty bastard about anything, he will keep his lips sealed, preferring to fight over divulging his secrets.

Death: If the Hero dies here, they respawn where they died.

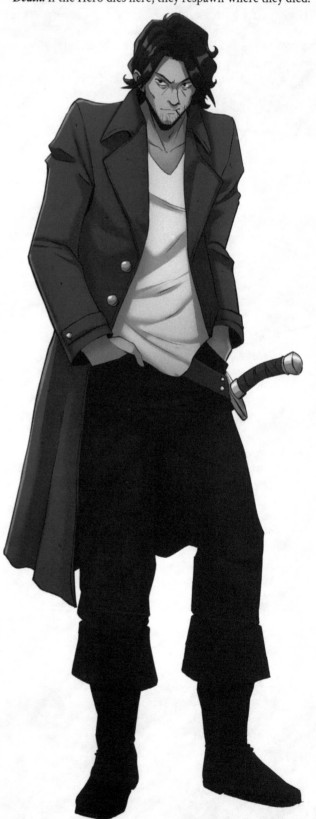

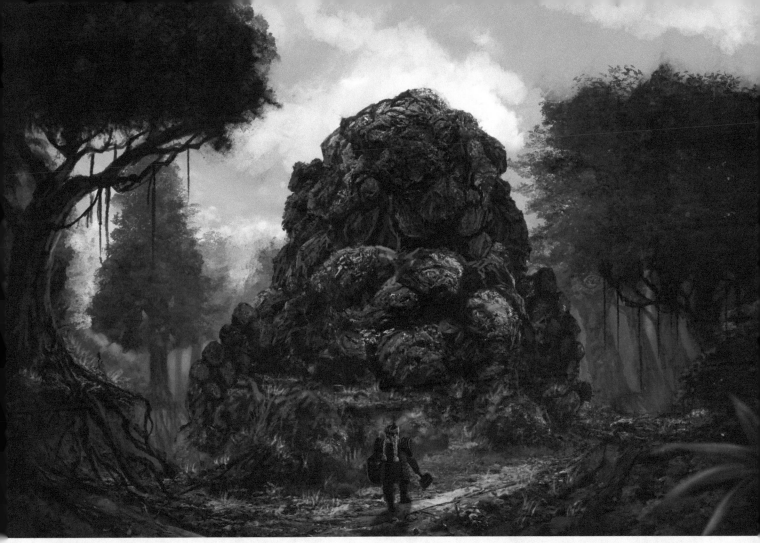

AREA 2: THE ROCKY HILL

Once the Hero has dealt with the dirty bastard, read the text box below:

> Continuing through the forest to the location marked on your map, you break through into a clearing. In the center, a giant hill of large, bleached stones is piled fifty feet high.
>
> Walking around the hill, you discover no gaps between the boulders. While you cannot see the top, you know there must be an entrance somewhere.

If the Hero uses Grabby Hands to touch the hill, they are unable to move any of the boulders. Trying to forcefully pry them away also proves fruitless, as the boulders are actually a giant stoned golem resting atop a hole in the ground where the crate is being kept.

Should a Hero use UV Light, there is no visible sign of magic. Only the hole below the stoned golem was created by magic, but that cannot currently be seen beneath it.

Working as an obstacle, a trap, and a protector, the stoned golem will not stir. So no matter what the Hero does, the only solution to wake it is to try climbing to the top of the hill.

Have the Hero make a Very Easy roll for the first half of the climb. On a successful roll of 2+, they ascend to the second half of the hill unharmed. On a failed roll, they fall, tumbling down the side of the hill for 1d4 damage and forcing them to roll to climb again.

If they make it to the top half of the hill, have them make another Very Easy roll. This time, if they fail, they take 1d8 damage and have to begin the climb again.

If the Hero is under the effects of the Potion of Enlargement, they can climb the hill in one roll instead of two. The damage they take from a failed roll will always only be 1d4 unless they die and the potion's effects wear off.

Once they make it to the top of the hill, they find nothing there but flat rock. A moment later, the hill begins to shift, causing them to make a Hard roll. On a successful roll of 5 or higher, the Hero makes it to the ground safely before the stoned golem is able to take form. If the Hero rolled a 4, they take 1d4 damage. If they rolled anything less, they take 1d8 damage unless they are under the effects of the Potion of Enlargement, in which case they would still only take 1d4 damage.

The stoned golem is absolutely massive and the main protector of the crate. Once it is standing at full height, the Hero can see the hole in the ground behind it. If they run for the hole, the golem will grab them and lift them into the air. Otherwise, it will not attack unless attacked first.

Multiple Heroes Modification: Regardless of how many Heroes are in the party, there will only be one stoned golem.

Role-Playing the Stoned Golem: Stoned golems speak miserably slowly and have patience for miles. They're also a bit spacey and tend to ramble. Stoned golems generally have a gentle disposition unless engaged in combat.

Unlike the dirty bastard, who is tight-lipped, the stoned golem loves to talk. Upon awakening from its slumber and facing the Hero, the first thing it says is, "Let me guess, you have come for Jokrana's treasure."

If asked who Jokrana is, the stoned golem will explain that she's an earth mage who hired the stoned golem to protect her treasure.

Should the Hero tell the stoned golem that the crate is stolen, it will not care, saying that humanoid squabbles are none of its business.

Being an earth mage, Jokrana is paying the stoned golem in delicious minerals that it cannot dig out of the soil on its own.

At some point, the stoned golem will talk about how it is oh so lonely and it has found pleasure in speaking to all the humanoids that have come to seek out the crate, even if it's had to kill them. It will reminisce about how one of the humanoids even shared a drink with it.

Have the Hero roll a Very Easy roll. A successful roll of 2 or higher will make the Hero believe that if they share a drink with the stoned golem, they might receive more favorable treatment. If more than one Hero is in the party, allow all Heroes to roll for this.

This can be any drink of the Hero's choice. The stoned golem will toast to a thousand years of good health, forgetting that most creatures don't live anywhere near that long.

After the stoned golem is done chatting the Hero up, they will reveal that the Hero must answer a riddle before they will be allowed access to the crate. If the Hero does not guess right on the first try and did not share a drink with the stoned golem, combat will immediately ensue. However, if the Hero did share a drink with the stoned golem, it will give them two chances to solve the riddle before attacking.

The stoned golem cannot be seduced as it has no interest in sex.

Below is the riddle that the Hero must answer to gain access to the crate:

> You stick your poles inside me. You tie me down to get me up. I get wet before you do. What am I?

The answer is a tent.

Should the Hero fail to answer correctly in their allotted number of times, they will have no choice but to fight the stoned golem. It's not meant to be beaten on the first try.

Stoned golems are notoriously slow. Though they have high Health Points, they can only attack once for every two times that the Hero attacks.

Death: If the Hero dies here, they respawn at the forest's edge in front of the stoned golem.

STONED GOLEM

Roll to Hit: 3+
Health Points: 22

Traits: Slow. The stoned golem only gets one combat action for every two the Hero gets.
Sex Style: None
Languages: Common, Golem

Description: A very lazy golem made out of stone. Because they suffer from the effects of psychoactive moss that grows on them, stoned golems are incredibly slow, both in speech and in action.

ATTACKS

Smash. Weaponless Attack: one target. *Hit:* (2d8) damage.

Stone Throw. *Ranged Weapon Attack:* one target. *Hit:* (1d8) ranged damage.

AREA 3: THE HOLE

Once the Hero has gotten past the stoned golem, they are free to explore the hole in the ground that Jokrana has created to hide her treasures. Read the boxed text below:

> An eight-foot wide crack in the ground looks down into a twelve-foot deep hole. The scent of death assaults your nose as you peer inside, finding a pile of dead bodies stacked around the crate. There are so many of them that you don't even need your rope to climb down.

Though slow, the stoned golem did its job well protecting the crate. All the bodies in the hole are of those who sought to steal the crate from Jokrana, meeting their untimely demise at the hands of the stoned golem.

If the Hero chooses to search around beneath the bodies, have them make a Normal roll. On a successful roll of 4 or higher, they find a long chest wedged between two bodies.

Before the Hero tries to open the chest, have them make a Hard roll. On a roll of 5 or higher, they can detect that the chest is trapped and will require a special action to open it. On a failed roll, the chest seems normal to them.

Should they fail the roll and attempt to open the chest, it will explode, destroying the loot inside and delivering 2d6 damage to the Hero.

If they passed the roll, choose one of the special scenarios below:

XXX – Using their connection with their Deity, the Hero can see that the chest will require sex magic to open it. To gain access to the treasure inside, the Hero must wear a blindfold and pleasure their Deity with their hands until the Deity is satisfied.

Multiple Heroes Modification: This sex act can be performed with any Hero in the party.

DRINK - Using their connection with their Deity, the Hero can see that the chest will require pouring a drink into their Deity's mouth without spilling a drop. This should be a one-ounce pour of liquor of the Hero's choice but can be substituted for 3 drinks of any other adult beverage.

Spilling any of the beverage will cause the chest to explode, destroying the loot inside and delivering 2d6 damage to the Hero.

Multiple Heroes Modification: Only one Hero will perform this action with the Deity. Should they fail, everyone standing in the hole takes damage.

BASE – The trap on the chest can be disarmed with a set of lockpicks and a successful Easy roll of 3 or higher. On a failed roll, the chest explodes, destroying the loot inside and delivering 2d6 damage to the Hero.

Multiple Heroes Modification: Everyone standing in the hole takes damage.

Inside the chest is a shortsword.

SHORTSWORD
Slot: Weapon
Type: One-Handed
Range: Close
Damage: 1d6

Death: If the Hero dies in the hole, they respawn outside of it.

SCENARIO 4: A TALE OF ICE

The fourth crate was taken high up The Naked Summit by the water mage Azad Khanna. He's hidden the crate in a trapped room inside the mountain. It will take the Hero navigating the small labyrinth to find the main chamber before they can disable the magic holding the crate prisoner. But first, they must find the hidden door on the side of the mountain.

You will notice that the map on the following page starts with the #2. That's because area 1 takes place outside the dungeon. Helping the Hero navigate this map might be difficult without a visual, as this dungeon is labyrinthine in nature. Therefore, it is recommended to draw out on a piece of paper for the Hero where they have already been so that they don't end up walking in circles.

AREA 1: THE CLIMB

At the start of this scenario, read the text box below:

> Your map leads you up the side of The Naked Summit, towering nearly 3,000 feet high and peeking into the clouds. Thankfully, you only had to climb three-quarters of the way up, but it's still high enough to hit snow.
>
> The ledge you're standing on is covered in ice, and a strong breeze threatens to blow you off the mountain at any moment. What's worse is there's no apparent entrance in the side of the rocky cliff where your map says there should be.

A fan of deception, Azad has placed three hidden doors in the side of the mountain. Only one grants entry into the dungeon. The other two are trapped.

More than likely, your Hero will search the area for an entrance. Have them roll a d6. On a Very Easy roll of 2 or more, they find Door #1.

On an Easy roll of 3 or more, they will find both Door #1 and Door #2. If they roll 5 or higher, they will find all three doors.

Should the Hero use UV Light, they will automatically find Door #2, as it is the only magical one.

If the Hero finds two or more doors during their search, give them the option of which one to open first.

Door #1 is trapped. Should the Hero try to open it, the door will explode. Regardless of where the Hero is standing, they will take 1d6 damage.

The explosion from the door knocks the ice loose from the other two doors, revealing Door #2 and Door #3, if the Hero hasn't found them already.

Door #2 is also trapped, though it is mostly meant to be a time waster. If the Hero chooses Door #2, follow the special scenario instructions below:

XXX – Using their connection with their Deity, the Hero can see that the door will require sex magic to open it. To open it, the Hero must have sex with their Deity in the lap dance position until the Hero is sexually satisfied. Once the sex act is completed, the door will open, revealing nothing but a rock wall on the other side.

Because of having to partially undress to perform the sex act, the Hero will also take 1d4 cold damage.

To do the lap dance position, the man sits on a straight-backed chair. The woman straddles him and sits on top, controlling the thrusting. He is not allowed to touch her throughout the entire act.

Multiple Heroes Modification: This sex act can be performed with any Hero in the party.

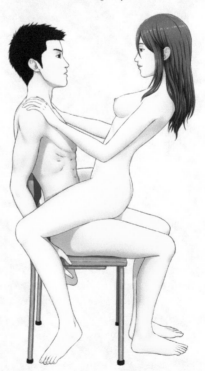

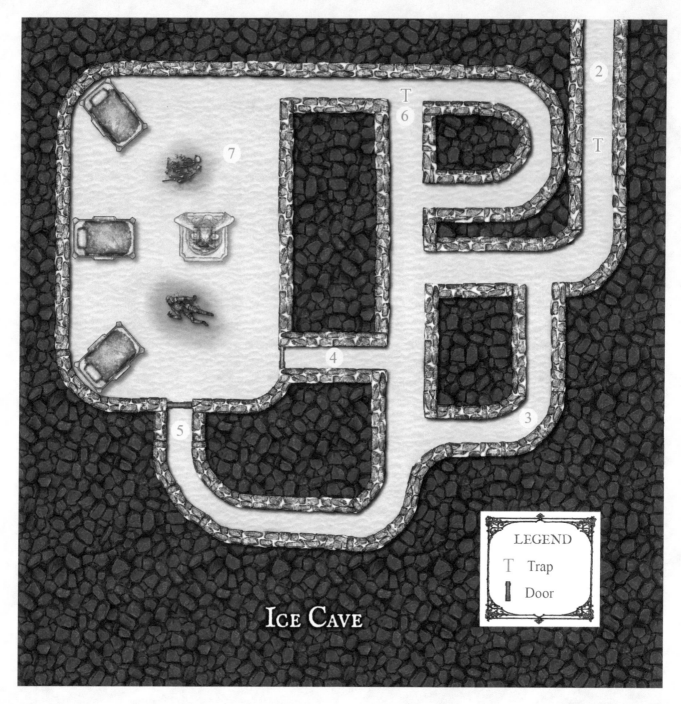

ICE CAVE

LEGEND

T Trap

▮ Door

DRINK - Using their connection with their Deity, the Hero can see that the door will require drinking a warming concoction to get it to open. This can be a one-ounce pour of Fireball, Peppermint Schnapps, or any other spicy liquor or liqueur. Alternatively, they can take three drinks of their favorite spicy or warm adult beverage. Mixed drinks that incorporate coffee and are served heated are perfect for this. For those who prefer beer, stouts and spiced or winter beers also work fine. Only the Hero needs to drink to open the door.

Once the drink has been taken, the door will open, revealing nothing but a rock wall on the other side.

Multiple Heroes Modification: Only one Hero is required to drink for this special scenario.

BASE – To open this door, the Hero will have to make a Very Hard roll. On a successful roll of 6, the door opens to reveal nothing but rock on the other side.

If the Hero fails the roll on the first try, they are not allowed to make it again. It does not matter that they cannot open the door, as it's not the right one anyway.

Multiple Heroes Modification: Each Hero is allowed to make this roll once.

Door #3 is the actual entrance into the mountain. It opens without protest, allowing the Hero inside.

Death: If the Hero dies on the mountain, they respawn in front of the doors.

Area 2: The Entrance

Once the Hero finds the real door, read them the text box below:

> The door opens to reveal an unlit corridor of unworked stone. Without a light source, you can't see very far down it. What you can see, however, is that the ground is covered in snow.

There are a lot of paths that the Hero can take once they venture further into the mountain. But first, they have to get past the scythe trap in this particular corridor.

If the Hero searches the area for the trap, finding it will require a Normal roll of 4 or higher. However, if they do not search the corridor, they will automatically trigger the trap, suffering 1d10 damage.

Once the Hero has passed the trap, use the map to guide them through the rest of the dungeon, describing the unmarked areas as best you can. Significant parts of the map have been given their own area guide.

Death: If the Hero dies in this corridor, they respawn outside, in front of the now open door.

Area 3: A Monster Encounter

If your Hero has chosen to take this path, they will come upon an ice vibrator.

Multiple Heroes Modification: Should your party have more than one Hero, add an ice vibrator for each party member.

ICE VIBRATOR

Roll to Hit: 4+
Health Points: 6

Traits: Night Vision
Sex Style: Vibrating Sex Toy
Languages: None

Description: A vibrating dildo made of ice that has gained sentience.

ATTACKS

Intense Vibrations. Weaponless Attack: one target. *Hit:* (1d4) damage.

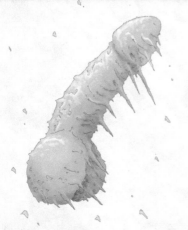

This particular foe can be seduced. Having sex with it will partially melt it, halving its Health Points and attack for the remainder of the combat. However, seducing it does not prevent combat, which will ensue after the sex act is completed.

To act out sex with the ice vibrator, the Hero must pleasure themselves with any vibrating sex toy until satisfaction has been achieved.

Area 4: The Wooden Door

This corridor dead ends at a wooden door. Though the locking mechanism is a bit complex, this is just a normal locked door. Using lockpicks or strength to get the door open will require a successful Hard roll of 5 or higher. On a failed roll, the Hero will not be allowed to roll again and will be forced to turn around and find another entrance into the chamber.

Area 5: The Steel Door

This corridor dead ends at a steel door. Read the special scenario rules below to discover how to open it:

XXX – Using their connection with their Deity, the Hero can see that the door will require sex magic to open it. To open it, the Hero must have sex with their Deity in the reverse bunny position until the Hero is sexually satisfied. Once the sex act is completed, the door will open.

To do the reverse bunny position, the man will lie prone on his back. The woman will straddle him backward, easing down until penetration is achieved. Then she will lower her torso toward his legs and make short, quick thrusts.

Multiple Heroes Modification: This sex act can be performed with any Hero in the party.

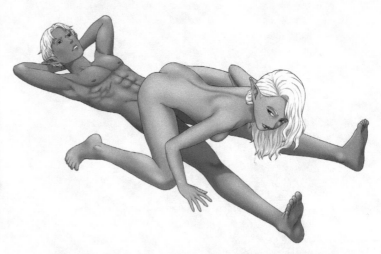

DRINK - Using their connection with their Deity, the Hero can see that the door will require drinking a warming concoction to open it. This can be a one-ounce pour of Fireball, Peppermint Schnapps, or any other spicy liquor or liqueur. Alternatively, they can take three drinks of their favorite spicy or warm adult beverage. d are perfect for this. For those who prefer beer, stouts and spiced or winter beers also work fine. Only the Hero needs to drink to open the door.

Multiple Heroes Modification: Only one Hero is required to drink for this special scenario.

BASE – There is no base version for opening this door. If your Hero would like to roll for it, allow them to, but no matter the outcome, they will not be able to open the door. If they happen to roll a 6, simply let them know that the door is solidly locked with seemingly no way inside.

AREA 6: THE PIT TRAP

No matter which direction your Hero comes from to get to this area, they will have to cross the pit trap to pass. If the Hero is searching for the trap, they can find it with a successful Very Easy roll of 2 or higher. If they do not search the area before entering, avoiding the trap requires a successful Hard roll of 5 or higher.

The pit is 10 feet deep, and anyone who falls into it will take 1d6 damage.

Climbing out of the trap requires a successful Very Easy roll of 2 or higher. On a fail, the Hero takes another 1d6 damage, divided by half, rounded down.

Death: If the Hero dies from falling in the pit trap, they will respawn on the other side of it, closest to area 6. If they decide to cross back over, they can easily avoid the trap.

AREA 7: THE ICE CHAMBER

Eventually, your Hero will find their way to this chamber. When they do, read the text box below:

You enter a massive chamber. The temperature in this room is several degrees colder than the winding corridors that brought you here.

In the center of the room is a giant sculpture made of ice depicting a human and an elf locked together in standing coitus. You can see the crate you seek encased inside the sculpture as well as a longbow.

Against the western wall, three queen size beds sit. While the heads of the beds are pushed against the wall, the feet all point toward the statue.

Two corpses stain the icy floor with their blood, one fresh, the other reduced to bones.

Using UV Light will reveal that the statue and beds are made of magic.

Should the Hero strike the statue with a weapon or spell, have them roll for damage. Whatever they roll gets reflected back at them.

If they try to damage the statue in another way, such as using fire to melt it, have them roll a 1d6 for damage against the statue. Whatever they roll is how much damage they will take.

Though their action results in injury to themselves, a small piece of ice chips off from the statue, revealing how to destroy it. Read the special scenario and decide how to proceed:

XXX – By examining the piece of statue, the Deity is able to determine that a series of sex magic is needed to destroy it.

Walking over to the bed furthest to the south, an image appears on the comforter of two lovers kissing. The first part of dispelling the magic is for the Deity to place an ice cube in their mouth, then kiss the Hero while sitting on the bed. The kiss can be as innocent or passionate as the Deity likes as long as the Hero can feel the coldness of their lips.

Once this is done, the statue will partially melt, birthing an icy heart into existence that will immediately initiate combat. Its stat block is after this Special Scenario box.

All icy hearts from this point on will share the same stat block. The icy hearts cannot be seduced.

After the icy heart is defeated, it will leave a small ice cube behind, revealing the next step in melting the statue.

The bedspread on the center bed will have changed, revealing the image of a man running an ice cube over a woman's breasts. To complete the next part, the Deity will have to take an ice cube and rub it over three erogenous zones of the Hero's body. Recommended areas are the nipples, the neck, the inner thighs, the stomach, the lips, or the genitals.

Once this act is performed, the statue will once again partially melt, birthing a second icy heart that the Hero will have to defeat. The icy heart will leave another ice cube behind to reveal the last act required to finish melting the statue.

After examining the ice cube, the comforter on the northern bed will change to reveal the image of a couple engaged in fellatio. To finally destroy the statue, the Deity will take an ice cube into their mouth, sucking on it until their mouth is very cold. Then they will perform oral sex on the Hero until the Hero is satisfied.

Once that is done, the statue will melt the rest of the way, allowing the Hero access to the crate and the longbow.

Should any of the above acts make either the Deity or the Hero uncomfortable, feel free to make a hybrid scenario by swapping it out with one of the other options in the DRINK or BASE section.

Required Props: Ice

Multiple Heroes Modification: If there is more than one Hero in your party, add an icy heart for every party member. Do this for every combat going forward in this scenario.

The Deity can delegate the various required sex acts in this special scenario to the Heroes in their party. The Deity does not need to be involved in them.

DRINK – By examining the piece of statue, the Deity is able to determine that destroying it will require imbibing a series of special drinks, each of which is specific to one of the beds.

Walking over to the bed furthest to the south, an image appears on the comforter of a glass with ice in it. The first part of dispelling the magic is for the Hero to drink a warming beverage over ice. This can be a shot of Fireball, Peppermint Schnapps, or any other spicy liquor or liqueur. If you do not have any of these in stock, anything over ice would be fine. For cocktails, the Hero only needs to take three sips.

Once this is done, the statue will partially melt, birthing an icy heart into existence that will immediately initiate combat.

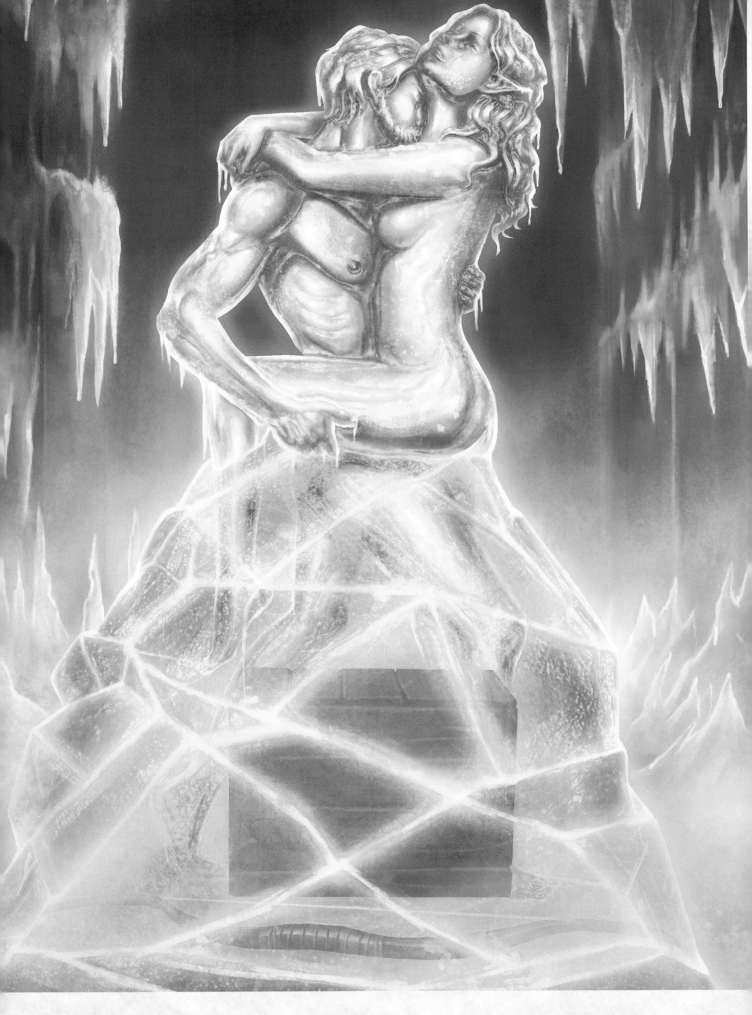

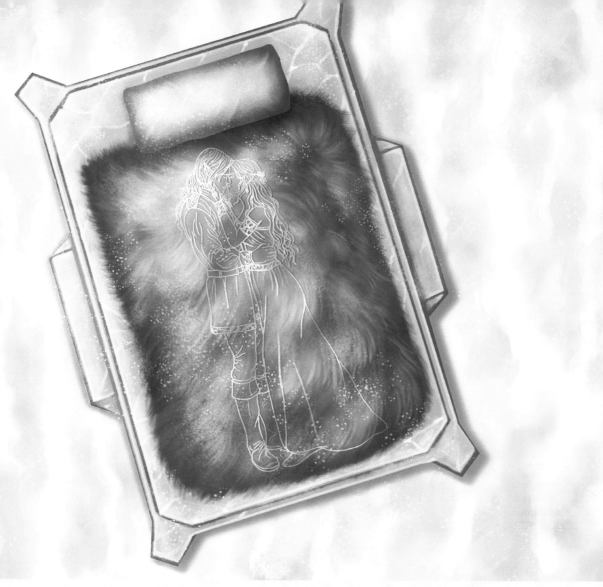

All icy hearts from this point on will share the same stat block. The icy hearts cannot be seduced.

After the icy heart is defeated, it will leave a small ice cube behind, revealing the next step in melting the statue.

The bedspread on the center bed will have changed, depicting a bottle. To complete the next part, the Hero will need to drink a Smirnoff Ice. If you do not have one on hand, taking any one-ounce pour of liquor or liqueur or three sips of any beverage will do.

Once this is done, the statue will once again partially melt, birthing a second icy heart that the Hero will have to defeat. The icy heart will leave another ice cube behind to reveal the last act required to finish melting the statue.

After examining the ice cube, the comforter on the northern bed will change to reveal a cocktail glass. To finally destroy the statue, the Deity will need to drink a Sex on a Snowbank cocktail. The recipe is provided after the icy heart monster stat block. If you cannot or do not want to make this beverage, taking any one-ounce pour of liquor or liqueur, or three sips of any beverage will do.

Once that is done, the statue will melt the rest of the way, allowing the Hero access to the crate and the longbow.

Multiple Heroes Modification: If there is more than one Hero in your party, add an icy heart for every party member. Do this for every combat going forward in this scenario.

A different Hero must drink for each bed. If there are only two Heroes in your party, then one of them must drink twice.

BASE – By examining the piece of statue, the Deity is able to determine that destroying it will require correctly answering a riddle while sitting on each bed.

Walking over to the bed furthest to the south, writing appears on the comforter. Read this riddle to the Hero. *What do men keep in their pants that their wives sometimes blow?* The answer is money. Coin is also acceptable.

If the Hero answers the riddle correctly, the statue will partially melt, and the riddle on the next bed will be revealed. However, if they should get the answer wrong, an icy heart will emerge from the statue and immediately initiate combat. Its stat block is after this scenario block.

This monster cannot be seduced. All icy hearts from this point on will share the same stat block.

Once the monster is defeated, the riddle on the next bed will be revealed. For the second bed, the riddle is as follows: *Every man has one; some are big, some are small. Blowing it feels great, but it will drip if you aren't careful. What is it?* The answer is a nose.

Again, if the Hero responds correctly, the statue will partially melt. Otherwise, they'll have to face and defeat another icy heart. Whichever occurs, the third riddle will be revealed on the comforter of the northernmost bed. Here it is: *What's a four-letter word that ends in "k" and means the same as intercourse?* The answer is talk.

After the final riddle is answered, the statue will melt the rest of the way, allowing the Hero access to the crate and the longbow.

Multiple Heroes Modification: Should there be multiple Heroes in your party, add an additional icy heart for each party member. Do this for every combat going forward in this scenario.

Your Heroes may collectively try to solve the riddles, but they are only allowed to submit one guess each time.

ICY HEART

Roll to Hit: 4+
Health Points: 13

Traits: Immune to melee damage. Can only receive damage from magic.
Sex Style: None
Languages: None

Description: Standing five feet tall and equally wide, this floating heart made of ice will freeze you from the inside out.

ATTACKS

Cold-Hearted. *Ranged Weapon Attack:* one target. *Hit:* (1d4) ranged damage.

SEX ON A SNOWBANK RECIPE

Ingredients:

- 1 ½ ounces Malibu rum
- 3 tablespoons Cream of Coconut
- 6 ice cubes

Instructions:

1. Place ingredients together in a blender.
2. Blend until smooth.
3. Pour into a glass and enjoy!

Once the statue is melted, the Hero can easily access the crate and the longbow. While they will have to return the crate to Famuhlel, the longbow is theirs to keep. The stats for it are below:

LONGBOW
Slot: Weapon
Type: Ranged
Damage: 1d8

Should the Hero want to continue exploring the dungeon, do not deter them. Though there is nothing else of note to find, half the fun is investigating.

Death: If the Hero dies in the chamber, have them respawn standing outside whatever door they used to enter.

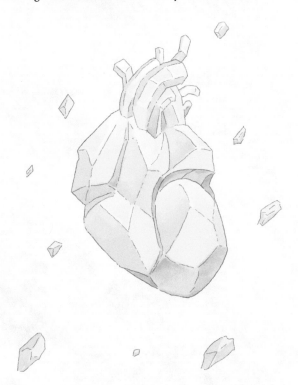

SCENARIO 5: A TALE OF LOSS

The final crate was taken by Urur Bilo, a known necromancer. Unfortunately, for him, before he could decipher the magic that was keeping the crate sealed, his hideout was raided by The Martyrs, a group of white mages whose purpose is to snuff out evil. Having found the crate and discerned it is of a sexual nature, they gave it to The Purists, who have tasked themselves with destroying all objects and magics sexual in nature. They have taken the crate to one of their temples to be disposed of. Little does the Hero know, they may be walking into a trap.

There is no map for this area.

AREA 1: OUTSIDE THE TEMPLE

When the temple comes into view, read the text box below:

Unlike the previous destinations on your map, this one takes you down a well-traveled path. You need not fear the monsters of the forest as an upward climb on a cart path leads you straight to a massive temple sitting atop a hill.

The view on both sides is stunningly beautiful. To the west, the temple looks out over farms and small villages in the distance, while the temple itself is a magnificent carved stone structure on the eastern side of the hill.

The door is open and clearly visible, the crate you seek only a short distance inside. You think claiming it will be a cakewalk until you hear a loud screeching noise overhead. When you look up, massive wings block out the sun, and you see sharp talons coming straight toward you.

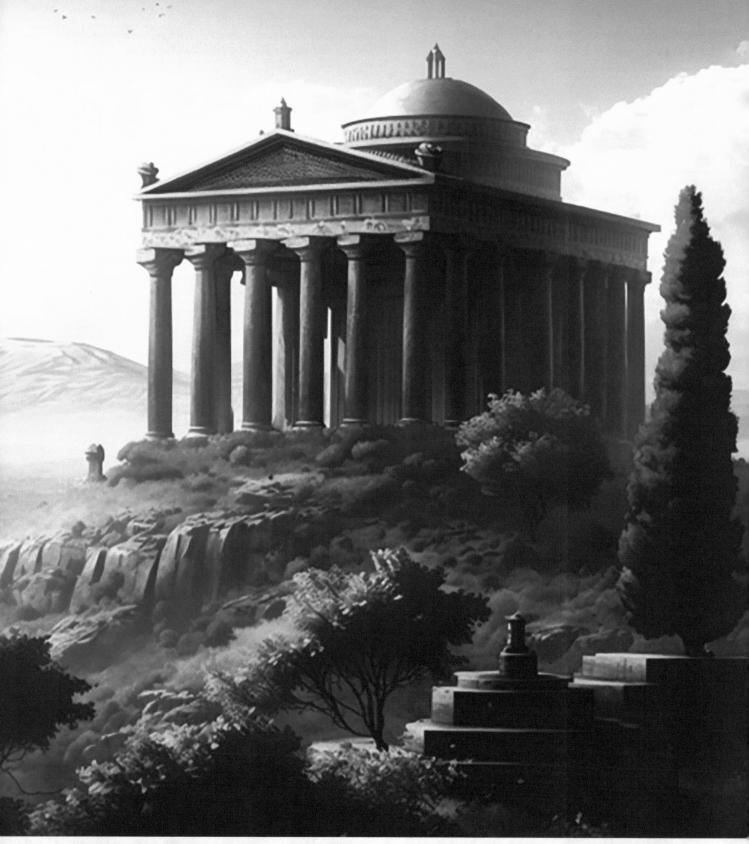

Before the Hero can reach the temple, they are set upon by a harpy.

Multiple Heroes Modification: If there is more than one Hero in the party, add an additional harpy for each Hero.

Have the Hero make a Hard roll. On a success of 5 or higher, they hear the harpy coming and will roll for Turn Order as normal. If they fail the roll, the harpy will catch them by surprise and automatically go first.

The harpy can be seduced, but it comes at the Hero's peril. Their sex style is clingy, which means they will clutch onto the Hero throughout the entire act. Only the male partner needs to reach climax for the act to conclude, as harpies only care about sex for the purpose of procreation. In a same-sex couple, the Deity role-playing the harpy must achieve climax.

HARPY

Roll to Hit: 5+
Health Points: 12

Traits: Flight. Harpies can only be hit with ranged attacks.
Sex Style: Clingy
Languages: None

Description: Half-human, half-bird, all aggression, these creatures swoop down from the sky to pick up their victims, carrying them back to their mountain nests where they mate with them before throwing them off a cliff.

ATTACKS

Talons. Weaponless Attack: one target. *Hit:* (1d6) damage.

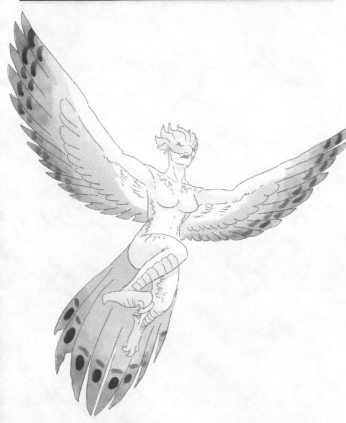

However, once the sex act is complete, the harpy will carry the Hero high up into the air and drop them, doing 1d20 damage.

Any Hero who runs to the temple for cover will meet a rude surprise when they attempt to enter. The door is trapped with magic, and anyone who tries to rush in will bounce right off it, sustaining 1d4 damage.

The door cannot be entered until the Hero has taken the time to read the engraving next to it, and unfortunately, they will not have time to do that until the harpy is dealt with.

Once the harpy is defeated, the Hero may approach the door to the temple. When they do, read the text box:

> As you approach the door to the temple, a plaque on the wall next to it catches your attention. The plaque reads: Learn. Play. Fight. You decide.

If the Hero did not try to enter the door during the harpy attack and they do so now, they will take 1d4 damage from the attempt.

Any Hero that uses UV Light before trying to go through the door can tell it is protected by magic.

If the Hero did not pick up on the clue from the plaque, inform them that they must decide whether they want to learn, play, or fight. If more than one Hero is in the party, this must be a group decision.

No matter how you have customized this campaign for the Hero so far, let them make this choice. They can always choose something else if they are not comfortable with the activity from their initial choice. Completing any of these will break the enchantment on the door, allowing them to enter the temple.

XXX (LEARN) – If the Hero chooses the Learn option, set a timer for 3 minutes. The Deity will teach the Hero how they enjoy being kissed. Then they will spend 3 minutes practicing. Once the timer is up, the shield will fade away from the door to the temple, making it passable.

Multiple Heroes Modification: All Heroes must be engaged to dispel the shield. If you have an even number of players split between the Deity and Heroes, divide them into pairs and perform this act simultaneously. If there is an odd number of players, the Deity will need to engage with two Heroes for 3 minutes each.

DRINK (PLAY) – If the Hero chooses the Play option, they will begin a drinking game. Both the Hero and the Deity should get either a beer, a mixed drink, or a glass of wine. No straight liquor.

Start the game by taking turns rolling a 1d10. The first player to roll a 3 is dubbed the Drunkard.

After that, each player will take turns rolling the die. The results will be as follows:

- When a 3 is rolled, the Drunkard takes a drink.
- When a 7, 8, or 9 is rolled, the person across from whoever rolled takes a drink.
- When a 10 is rolled, both the Hero and the Deity drink.
- When a 4 or 1 is rolled, both players must place their thumb on top of the table. Whoever is last to do this drinks.
- For any other numbers rolled, no one drinks.

The game continues until either the Hero or the Deity has finished their drink, at which point the shield will fade away from the door to the temple, making it passable.

Multiple Heroes Modification: All Heroes should participate in the drinking game. The game ends when either one of the Heroes or the Deity finishes their drink.

In games with an uneven number of players, when a 7, 8, or 9 is rolled, the person who rolled gets to choose who drinks.

BASE (FIGHT) – If the Hero chooses the Fight option, a ball of purged perversions is spawned and must be defeated. Only one of these monsters is spawned, no matter how many Heroes are in the party.

The ball of purged perversions cannot be seduced. Its stat block is below.

Once the monster is defeated, the shield will fade away from the door to the temple, making it passable.

Death: If the Hero dies in this area, they will respawn in front of the temple.

BALL OF PURGED PERVERSIONS

Roll to Hit: 3+
Health Points: 19

Traits: Night Vision
Sex Style: None
Languages: None

Description: A massive ball of sex toys and genitals, this monster is straight from your perverted nightmares.

ATTACKS

Assault. Weaponless Attack: one target. *Hit:* (1d8) damage.

AREA 2: INSIDE THE TEMPLE

Once the Hero enters the temple, read the boxed text:

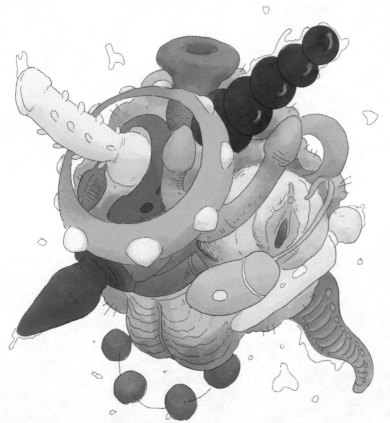

The inside of the temple is absolutely massive, with a 50-foot high ceiling and large stone columns supporting the roof. At the back of the room is a giant statue of Asheia, Goddess of Purity. Before it, the crate you seek sits in a large glass box.

The walls are painted with murals of Asheia blessing the people of The Unbound Domain, cleansing them of their impure thoughts. Four copper braziers decorate the room's corners, though they are currently unlit. Light streams in through stained-glass windows near the ceiling, painting the room in a mosaic of color.

Getting the crate out of the glass box will be much easier said than done, as the box is made of magic. A Hero who uses UV Light in the room will know this immediately. They will also be able to see the hidden message on the glass box, which speaks of how dispelling the magic will require making a sacrifice to each of the braziers in the room.

If the Hero should choose to attack the glass box, any damage dealt to it will be reflected back at them. However, attacking the box will reveal the secret message inscribed in it, telling them that they will have to sacrifice to each of the braziers to dispel the magic keeping the crate captive.

Should the Hero try to lift the glass box, it is too heavy, and they cannot move it.

Regardless of which brazier the Hero chooses to investigate first, the message remains the same. They must choose one item from their inventory and cast it into the brazier. Once they do this, the brazier will light up, and the glass box will flash.

The next brazier will ask them to sacrifice a weapon. After they toss their weapon of choosing into the brazier, a fire will bloom inside it. The glass box will flash, indicating that the sacrifice has been accepted.

The third brazier will demand a sacrifice of magic. To satisfy this, the Hero must choose a Unlimited spell to permanently forget. Once they have sacrificed a spell of their choosing, the brazier will light up, and the box will flash.

The final brazier requires the sacrifice of a Limited spell. After the sacrifice has been made, the last brazier will light up, and the glass box will disappear from around the crate.

Before the Hero has a chance to collect the crate, a man enters the room. This is Nhasein Pummo, a Purist who has been sent to destroy the crate.

When the Hero goes to retrieve the crate, read the boxed text below:

Just as you lay your hands on the crate, a voice speaks behind you. "Judging by the light in the braziers, it's probably safe to assume that you didn't come here to worship."

As you turn, you see a dark-skinned male gnome wearing white standing just inside the temple entrance. Judging by his attire and the disapproving look on his face, you surmise that he is a Purist—a destroyer of all things perverted.

"However, the Goddess teaches us to know the measure of truth before casting judgment on others," the Purist continues. "So tell me, what is your truth? Why are you here?"

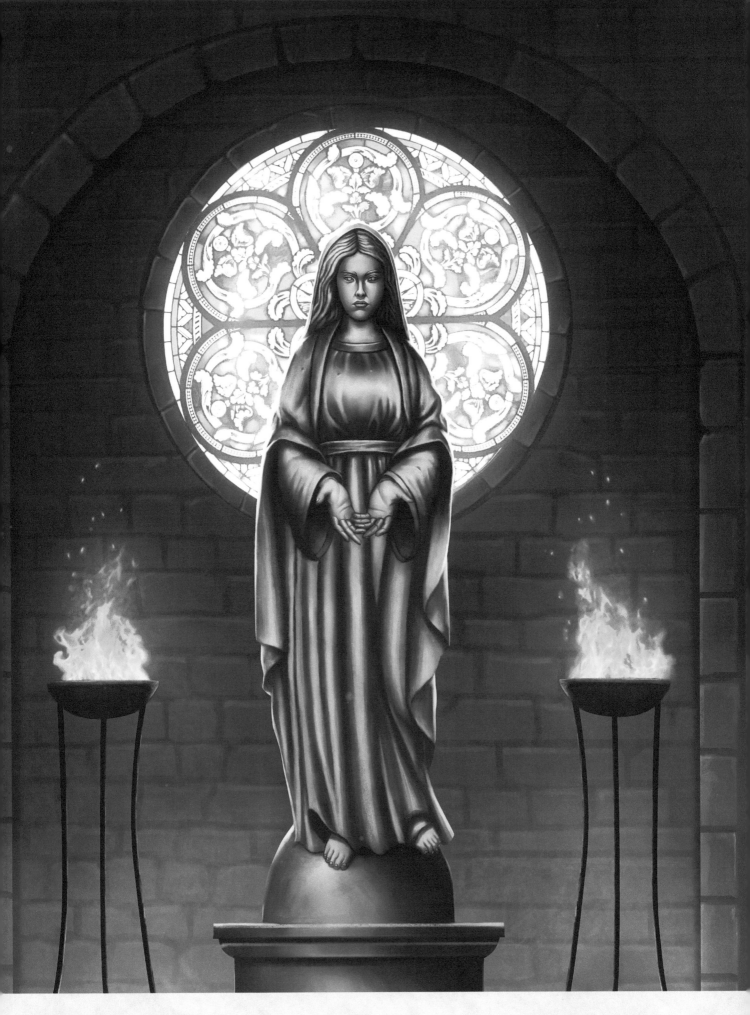

The Hero now has a chance to respond to the accusations of thievery. If the Hero tells Nhasein the truth, he will allow them to leave with their life as long as they abandon the crate. Otherwise, combat will ensue. Being a Purist and against all things perverted, Nhasein cannot be seduced. His stat box is below.

Multiple Heroes Modification: No matter how many Heroes are in the party, there is only one Nhasein Pummo.

Alternatively, the Hero can choose to lie. If they say something along the lines of that they were sent by other Purists to relocate the crate, the Deity should make a Normal roll to see if Nhasein believes them. On a successful roll of 4+, Nhasein will allow the Hero to take the crate. If the roll fails, Nhasein will not believe the Hero, and combat will ensue.

NHASEIN PUMMO

Roll to Hit: 4+
Health Points: 30

Traits: None
Sex Style: None
Languages: Common

Description: A Purist sent to destroy Famuhlel's crate in the Temple of Asheia.

ATTACKS

Stone Throw. *Ranged Weapon Attack:* one target. *Hit:* (1d6) ranged damage.

Purify. Limited Spell: one target.

PURIFY

Requirements: Must be able to speak and move hands.
Type: Limited
Range: Ranged
Description: Removes a Cummancer's ability to cast all sex magic, including both Unlimited and Limited spells, forcing them to switch to regular weapons until their next death. Only Purists can learn this spell.

Nhasein is very powerful and not meant to be defeated on the first try. For his first action, he will cast Purify, which will force the Hero to use regular melee and ranged weapons. Every time the Hero dies, Nhasein will use his first action to cast Purify again.

Once Nhasein is defeated, the braziers will flame brightly, and the Hero will gain the knowledge of how to perform the Limited spell Sleep Spray.

SLEEP SPRAY

Requirements: Must be able to see and move hands.
Type: Limited
Range: Ranged
Description: You spray a liquid concoction of sleep chemicals on your opponent, putting them to sleep. If the foe takes damage or you leave the room they're in, they wake

back up. If you attack a sleeping enemy, you do not need to Roll to Hit.

Death: If the Hero dies in this area, they will respawn in area 1, outside the temple door.

END OF CAMPAIGN RESULTS

Once the Hero has returned the crates to Famuhlel, they may choose one of the following items or upgrades. However, if they do not bring all 5 crates back with them, they will have failed the quest, and she will not reward them.

If asked what is in the crates, Famuhlel will respond by saying, "Trust me, telling you would only put you in more danger."

MAGICAL THONG
Slot: Bottoms
Type: Armor
Description: Allows the Hero to have and use an additional Limited spell.

PLAY WITH FIRE (SPELL)
Requirements: Must be able to see and move hands.
Type: Unlimited
Range: Ranged
Description: Allows you to manipulate any source of fire in an area you can see. This includes spreading the fire by up to five feet in one direction, making it grow smaller or go out, and changing the shape. While you can use this spell to barricade small areas, it cannot be used as an attack. Creatures who step through this fire will take 1d4 damage. This spell is limited to one casting per area.

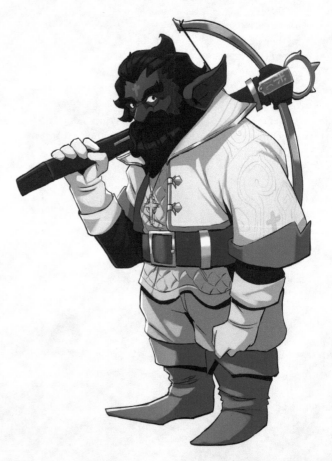

BROTHEL TICKET

Description: This ticket entitles the owner to one trip to the Hadel Brothel. See the Hadel Brothel section on the following page for instructions.

If there is more than one Hero in the party, each Hero is allowed to choose a reward. Heroes are allowed to select the same reward as others.

This is the end of this campaign. If you are interested in experiencing more Lewd Dungeon Adventures, please sign up for our mailing list to know when the next adventure will be available. https://www.subscribepage.com/lewd

You can also support us on Patreon for behind the scenes info on the artwork for the series as well as to gain early access to campaigns currently being written: https://www.patreon.com/lewddungeonadventures

HADEL BROTHEL

The Hadel Brothel offers the finest in adult entertainment that Hadel has to offer. Anyone with a brothel ticket may visit the brothel once and choose from a selection of 3 playmates. The gender of each character is referred to as them, and the Deity is to act the character out as their own gender.

SARQEN THE PERFECTIONIST

Race: Elf
Personality: Confident
Description: Sarqen has always had an obsession with sex, making it their life goal to be the ultimate lover. They pride themselves on meeting the needs of every client that purchases their services. Well-versed in all things love-making, they never quit until their client is lying exhausted in a heap of their own pleasure-juices.

To role-play Sarqen, the Deity will go above and beyond to meet every request the Hero has, giving maximum effort to the act. The Brothel Ticket entitles the Hero to one orgasm from Sarqen. Holding themselves in high regard, once the Hero has climaxed, Sarqen will demand that they pay more if they want continued servicing.

DULDOHR THE DOMINANT

Race: Dwarf
Personality: Controlling
Description: Duldohr was sold into slavery as a child and lived doing the bidding of others until they were traded to the Hadel Brothel to pay off a debt. With the brothel's madam giving them sexual freedom, Duldohr decided to reclaim their power by vowing never to take orders from anyone again, except for the madam, of course.

When a Hero hires Duldohr, the dwarven prostitute calls all the shots. Where people used to use them, they now use their clients for their own selfish pleasure. Whether the client gets off or not is none of Duldohr's concern. People come from all over the land to relinquish control to the liberated dwarf.

To role-play Duldohr, the Deity may make any demands they want from the Hero. If the Hero refuses to comply with anything Duldohr wants, then they forfeit the remainder of their time at Hadel Brothel.

While Duldohr is dominant, they are not sadistic. All sex acts should be about Duldohr receiving the most pleasure, using the Hero as a simple tool to achieve climax. Duldohr is very vocal about what they want, will make demands, and give instructions for adjustments if the Hero is not doing things to their liking.

NHADAM THE ASS MASTER

Race: Human
Personality: Quirky
Description: Nhadam has one specialty and obsession. Butt play. Whether it be by using toys or body parts, Nhadam is all about exploring the rim. They equally enjoy both giving and receiving pleasure in this manner.

Nhadam will be willing to collaborate with the Hero on how the session will go. While the majority should be about anal, they will honor up to two requests for other activities. However, they will perform these acts without enthusiasm. If the Hero makes a third request, Nhadam will terminate the session.

Multiple Heroes Modification: Should multiple Heroes choose the Hadel Brothel option, only the Deity may act out the role of the prostitutes. Heroes may choose to share the same prostitute simultaneously or take their turns individually. Alternatively, they may each choose a different prostitute.

SEX ACTS FOR HERO DEATHS

When a Hero dies, use the chart on the following page and a d6 to determine what act needs to be performed to resurrect them. Unless timed, all acts must be carried out to the Deity's satisfaction.

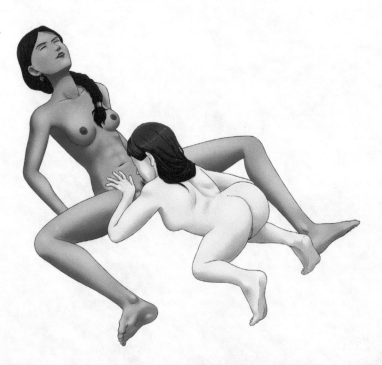

1 – Deity's choice. The Deity will pick the sex act to be carried out.

2 – Manual stimulation (a handjob or fingering) for 3 minutes.

3 – Backward Bounce position.

4 – Oral Stimulation (a blowjob or cunnilingus) for 3 minutes.

5 – Wall Banger position.

6 – Hero's choice. The Hero will pick the sex act to be carried out.

Below is a description of the Backward Bounce and Wall Banger positions.

For the sake of ease, the descriptions of these sex acts were written with a man and a woman in mind. If the position is not applicable to your gender, please sub it out with something more appropriate or the drinking version of the game. The same applies if the idea of performing one of these sex acts makes you uncomfortable or you are not physically able.

POSITION: BACKWARD BOUNCE

Location: On a bed

Description: Male partner sits on a bed, angled back and propped up on his hands. The woman straddles him backward, lowering herself and curling her knees. She initiates penetration, then bounces on the man's lap.

POSITION: WALL BANGER

Location: Against a wall

Description: Female partner stands facing a wall. She arches over ever so slightly and presses her hands against the wall. The male partner comes from behind, initiating penetration. He places his hands on her waist while controlling the thrusting.

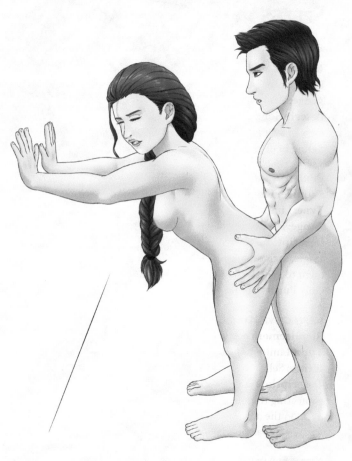

BASE ACTS FOR HERO DEATHS

Should the Hero and/or Deity be in a refractory period and not wish to imbibe in alcohol, the following acts may be used for Hero resurrection. Use the chart below and a d6 to determine what act needs to be performed.

1 – Deity's choice. The Deity will pick the act to be carried out.

2 – The Hero must tell the tale of a fearsome monster they faced.

3 – The Hero must sing or hum the chorus from *Toss a Coin to Your Witcher*.

4 – The Hero must take a picture of something in the room.

5 – The Hero must skip around the table 3 times.

6 – The Hero must take 3 drinks of water.

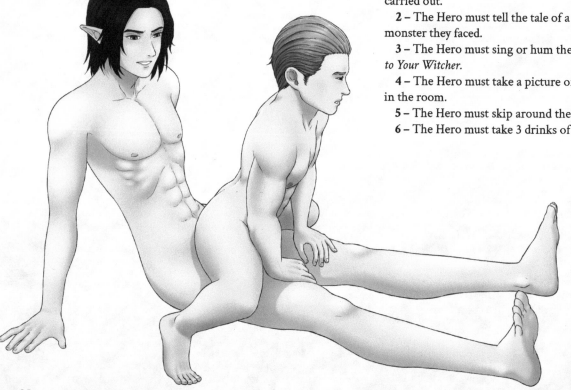

Spells in This Campaign

Bad Touch

Requirements: Must be able to move hands.
Type: Unlimited
Range: Ranged
Description: Ethereal hands form to touch a target within view in every uncomfortable way imaginable. The sheer feeling of disgust does 1d8 damage to the soul.

Purify

Requirements: Must be able to speak and move hands.
Type: Limited
Range: Ranged
Description: Removes a Cummancer's ability to cast all sex magic, including both Unlimited and Limited spells, forcing them to switch to regular weapons until their next death. Only Purists can learn this spell.

Reflective Barrier

Requirements: Must be able to speak.
Type: Limited
Range: Self
Description: A thick rubber barrier forms around the caster, protecting them from 3 damage and reflecting that damage back on the attacker. The effects of this spell last for the entire combat, and casting it requires an action.

Sleep Spray

Requirements: Must be able to see and move hands.
Type: Limited
Range: Ranged
Description: You spray a liquid concoction of sleep chemicals on your opponent, putting them to sleep. If the foe takes damage or you leave the room they're in, they wake back up. If you attack a sleeping enemy, you do not need to Roll to Hit.

Splash Guard

Requirements: Must be able to speak.
Type: Unlimited
Range: Self
Description: You make an upward wave of your hands, causing a thin sheet of plastic to rise before you. The splash guard will protect you against half of any incoming magic damage you would have otherwise taken from an attack until the end of your next turn. It does not protect against melee damage. This spell must be cast before the damage is received.

Special Thanks

The Lewd Dungeon Adventures team would like to thank the following people for helping to bring this project to life: P.A.L., D&M, Rob 2.0, 8bitgirl, Tim Ã–., AaronM, Inquisitor Abes, Aeriwyna, Ross Asbill, Ass5000, Raph B, Keenbo Babino, Mark Bacon, Murphy Barrett, Raphael Bartholdi, bluephyr, Jordan Blythe, Patrick Boehme, Donald "Jokermun" Boyd, Jeremy Brown, Merritt Smith & Laura Byard, Citizen Cain, PhD, Marcus Cairne, Bryce Leland Carlson, Alfio Cavassa, Benoit Cecyre, Celtric, The Chemistress, Jay Cloud, Cnayur, Menachem Cohen, Con3Ras, Jason Criscuolo, Jase D, Aaron D, Bec & Dan, Dannon, Daximus, Sasha Dean, Madeleine Dile, discoursian, Dragondarium, Llullana & Durion, Michelle E, Darren & Christy Ehlers, Ekdesr, ELF, Emiel, Entayan, Cris F, Keith Fannin, Feronus, Mt Flower, Alex Fosth, Fym, Diacast gaming, Darrell Garcia, Gargelspouzel, Ryan George, Soft Ghoulll, Jim Glass, GNeo808, Koenraad Gossaert, Kirk Graves, Stuart Grosse, Gyshi, Seth Hartley, Jason and Robin Hasty, Tom Henson Jr, Charli-Anne Horton, icephoenix, David Benito Iglesias, IronChefBoyardee, Isilian, M en J, Josh & Joann, Tyler Johnson, Kage, THE Kevin, Lady Kiiri, KireWithe, Kothar, M. A. LaMothe, Lebis, Craig Levengood, T.N. Liput, Lord and Lady Lionel and Lara Longcock, Loopylou, Lorisia, Rob Lowry, Nate Lyon, Gracie M, Stan The Man, Paul Marzagalli, Mastertoenail, Guy Matte, Matthew, Stephen McCabe, David "Chartan" McFall, MichellelovesCarlos, Mikailos, Chaos & Mischief, Shima Mizuki, mj_and_hj, Berny Molina, Poet and Muse, Nekosluagh, Neuros, Ted Nox, Kalon Ohmstede, Logan Ondzik, Aljinon Padgnus, Rob Paine, Timothy Bove (Paladin), Jafo the Panda, PappiBoardGames, Joseph S. Perry, Brian David Phillips, Scooby Phoenix, Danger Pixies, Jose' Placeres, Headless Hydra Press, Phil Preston, Martin Prucha, Pumpkin, RadCat, Rarzilla, Kaidan Redgrave, RobertLisa, Philip W Rogers Jr, Richard "Damoncord" Rudel Jr, S, Josh S., Mike Sanders, Michael Santana, scorpione40, Steven "Feral" Scott, Selmis, Shazam_XLT, Mister Sheep, Sheika, Mark A. Siefert, Pepe Silvia, Sledge, Smiley, "filkertom" Tom Smith, André Sommer, Spacecase, Squirrel, Starlion, Starocotes, StrikerPrince, Adam Strutt, Stuart, The Tabaxi, Kenneth Tedrick, By The Tentacles, Thanay, Trey, Michael Tritt, Seb Tudor, V, Kawthir & Valette, Valhollar, Velrissa, Russell Ventimeglia, Kenzo W, Dan Wallace, Wayne, Greg Weeks, Wesley, Ian Whitehead, Wolframsmith, Ryder Frankle and Red Shark Minis, The Sid XXX, Zantaraz